WEIGHT LOSS UNVEILED: YOUR GUIDE TO A HEALTHIER YOU

THELMA K. WHITE

INTRODUCTION

Many people set out on the path to weight loss with vigor and optimism. It's a path that has the promise of a happier and healthier future along with difficulties and victories. The measures you take to lose those excess pounds and adopt a way of life that promotes general wellbeing will be guided, accompanied, and informed by this book.

Why Weight Loss Is Important

Losing weight is much more than just looking good or fitting into smaller clothes. Regaining your health and vigor is the goal. Numerous health concerns, including heart disease, diabetes, and joint problems, can be brought on by being overweight. You're putting less stress on your body by losing weight, giving yourself the best chance to live a longer, more active life.

Setting Realistic Objectives

Setting realistic objectives is crucial as you start this adventure. While quick changes could make for interesting entertainment, lasting improvements take time in the real world. Your trip is special, and your objectives should show that. Setting attainable goals that acknowledge your progress along the road is essential, whether your goal is to lose a big amount of weight or just a few obstinate pounds.

There is no one-size-fits-all method for losing weight. It's about figuring out what suits you, your body, and your way of life the best. This book will teach you about the science of weight loss, how to develop healthy behaviors, and how to get past challenges. But keep in mind that the journey itself is just as important as the final goal.

Encouraging Change

Although it can be frightening, change is what spurs progress. Approach this journey with an open mind and a desire to learn as you go out on it. You'll learn that weight loss is a process that includes mental, emotional, and even spiritual growth in addition to the physical aspects. In order to embrace change, you must let go of old behaviors that no longer serve you and make room for new ones that improve your wellbeing.

A Holistic Strategy

This book approaches weight loss holistically. It involves more than just sticking to a strict diet and doing vigorous exercise. It involves being aware of the science underlying weight management, establishing appropriate eating habits, including frequent exercise, and cultivating an optimistic outlook. You're putting yourself in a position to succeed on many fronts by taking care of all these factors.

Your Path, Your Journey

Recall that this is your adventure as you read the ensuing chapters. You are in charge and have the ability to decide according to your values and ambitions. Although there may be ups and downs, each step you take will bring you closer to the healthier, happier version of yourself.

So let's start. Turn the page to begin your journey to a lighter, brighter, and more colourful you, then plunge into the chapters that lie ahead. Keep in mind that you're not walking this route alone. You can find the knowledge, inspiration, and resources you need in this book to be successful. Prepare yourself to learn the secrets of long-lasting weight loss and to adopt a lifestyle that supports your body, mind, and spirit. Your journey has just begun.

Chapter 1

UNDERSTANDING WEIGHT LOSS

Knowledge acts as the compass and the map in the complex web of weight loss. Understanding the underlying science governing how our bodies regulate weight is essential for successfully navigating this journey. The mysteries behind weight loss will be revealed in this chapter, which delves deeply into the function of calories, the intricacies of metabolism, and the variety of body fat. You'll obtain a thorough understanding of the dynamics at work and be equipped to make wise choices on your path to change by looking at these key ideas.

The Study of Calories

The unit of exchange in the world of weight management is the calorie. These food-derived energy units control the delicate balance between weight increase, maintenance, and decrease. The idea is straightforward: weight gain occurs when you ingest more calories than your body uses, whereas weight loss occurs when you burn more calories than you take in.

But not every calorie is made equal. It is important to choose foods that offer the best nutrition per calorie when considering nutrient density. Vitamin, mineral, and fiber-rich foods nourish and energize your body, boosting your overall health as you work towards a healthier weight.

Demystifying Metabolism

The body's engine, or metabolism, is a dynamic system of chemical interactions that maintains life. It is in charge of transforming food into the energy required for physical activities and biological functions. Your body burns calories while at rest, or at its basal metabolic rate (BMR), which is a baseline characteristic that affects how you control your weight.

Contrary to popular belief, lifestyle decisions have a big impact on how our metabolism functions. Regular exercise, especially strength training, can increase your muscle mass and raise your BMR. Your metabolism might also be impacted by the frequency and make-up of your meals. Instead of eating a few substantial meals throughout the day, spreading calories out among several smaller ones can aid in sustaining a steady energy expenditure.

Various forms of body fat

Body fat has many different forms, each of which has effects on health. It is not a single entity. Under the skin, subcutaneous fat serves as a source of energy. Visceral fat, on the other hand, encloses key organs and poses greater health hazards. Insulin resistance, inflammation, and an increased risk of chronic diseases including diabetes and cardiovascular problems are all linked to excess visceral fat.

For complete weight loss and increased health, it's crucial to target both visceral and subcutaneous fat. While visceral fat must be addressed holistically, including cardio and strength training along with dietary alterations, subcutaneous fat may respond more noticeably to food changes and exercise.

Putting what is learned into practise

With knowledge of calories, metabolism, and body fat, you are now prepared to make wise choices as you embark on a weight loss journey. Keep in mind that this journey involves more than just weight loss or gain; it's a complete makeover aimed at improving your general wellbeing. You'll not only reach your weight reduction objectives by making progressive, lasting changes to your food and lifestyle, but you'll also pave the way for a healthier future.

You will learn more about creating a balanced nutrition plan, creating an efficient training routine, and cultivating a positive mindset as you read the chapters that follow. This chapter sets the basis, giving you the background information required to comprehend and appreciate the changes occurring inside your body. Accept the process, keep learning, and let your newly acquired knowledge lead you to long-lasting success—a success that includes not only weight loss but also increased vigour and a renewed feeling of self.

Chapter 2

BUILDING A STRONG FOUNDATION

Building a solid foundation is essential in the complex tapestry of weight loss. The goal of this foundation is to create a sustainable and nourishing eating strategy that supports your body's needs while advancing you towards your weight loss objectives. It goes beyond simple dieting. The skill of developing a balanced meal plan, the relevance of portion control, and the acceptance of nutrient-rich foods are all explored in this chapter. You may create a harmonious relationship with food that not only promotes weight loss but also improves your general wellbeing by learning these essential concepts.

Developing a Balanced Dietary Plan

A balanced diet is an orchestra of tastes, nutrients, and nourishment that supports your efforts to lose weight and improve your health. This strategy encourages you to include a wide variety of nutrient-rich foods in your meals and celebrates diversity. It is about a flexible framework that supports your body's nutritional needs rather than strict regulations.

Introduce a variety of vibrant fruits and vegetables to your diet to start. The vitamins, minerals, and antioxidants in these colorful foods help your immune system, skin health, and general vigor. Muscle growth and repair depend heavily on lean proteins, whether they come from animal or plant sources. Whole grains, root vegetables, and legumes include complex carbs that offer sustaining energy for your everyday activities.

Using portion control to navigate

Portion control acts as a compass to help you navigate the calorie consumption seas. It's an awareness exercise that teaches you to discern when you've had enough without succumbing to overindulgence. The propensity for large amounts in our culture has contributed to the rise of obesity. You regain control over your intake by being aware of proper serving sizes.

Visual signals can be effective portion control allies. A portion of carbs should be around the size of your closed fist, but a dish of protein should be about the size of your palm. To make sure you're getting a range of nutrients and fibre, cover half of your plate with veggies. Pay attention to your body's hunger and fullness cues and let them direct your eating habits.

The nutrient-dense bounty

The gems in the weight reduction crown are foods high in nutrients. These meals provide a lot of important nutrients, frequently condensed into a relatively little package of calories. By including them in your diet, you're supplying your body with the nutrients it needs to thrive while simultaneously promoting weight loss.

Kale and spinach are two examples of dark leafy greens that are rich in calcium, iron, and vitamins A, K, and C. Berries are dazzling sources of antioxidants that fight oxidative damage and inflammation. Omega-3 fatty acids, which are essential for heart health and brain function, are found in fatty seafood like salmon and mackerel. Nuts and seeds provide your food with a delicious crunch, wholesome lipids, and fiber.

Keeping Indulgence and Nutrition in Check

Finding the right balance between feeding your body and indulging in life's joys is essential to the weight loss journey. Total restriction frequently results in resentment and disobedience, whereas a mindful indulgence mindset might promote a healthier relationship with food.

Be careful of your actions when you treat yourself to indulgent foods. Take in the flavors, textures, and scents by using all of your senses. You may thoroughly enjoy the event while still having control over your decisions when you indulge mindfully. Keep in mind that enjoying goodies as a part of your journey is more important than banning them.

A Gastronomic Journey

By adopting the practise of laying a solid nutritional foundation, you're starting a gastronomic journey that feeds the body and the soul. The framework for your change is built with a focus on nutrient-rich meals, portion control, and a balanced eating plan. This chapter focuses on developing a mentality and eating style that will benefit you far beyond your weight reduction objectives rather than just what you put on your plate. You'll study the areas of exercise and fitness, mentality, and healthy behaviours as you continue your journey through the remaining chapters, strengthening this foundation as you move closer to being a healthier and more vibrant version of yourself.

Chapter 3

EXERCISE AND FITNESS

Exercise stands out as a colorful thread that runs through every aspect of your transformation in the dynamic fabric of weight loss. It involves developing a lifestyle that values movement, vitality, and empowerment rather than just changing your body. This chapter launches a thorough investigation into the complex world of fitness and exercise, exploring the subtleties of creating a successful workout routine, revealing the mutually beneficial relationship between cardiovascular and strength training, appreciating the value of regular movement, and fostering a positive attitude towards exercise. Engaging in exercise will take your entire being to new levels of strength and well-being, taking you on a journey that goes beyond weight reduction.

Creating a Successful Workout Programme: Your Individual Blueprint

Think of your exercise regimen as a personal road map that shows how to become a stronger, healthier version of yourself. It's a strategic plan created to support your goals and take into account your particular body and preferences, not just a collection of random activities. Clarify your fitness objectives before lacing up your trainers. Are muscle gain, increased endurance, weight loss, or a combination of these goals your main goals?

You should incorporate both cardiovascular and strength training into your exercise programme. Cardiovascular exercises raise your heart rate, boost your calorie burn, and improve your mood by releasing endorphins. These can involve exercises like jogging, cycling, swimming, or brisk walking. On the other side, strength training is essential for developing lean muscle mass, which not only improves your appearance but also accelerates your resting metabolic rate.

Strength training vs. Cardiovascular Training: A Harmonious Fusion

Although cardiovascular and strength training might seem like two separate disciplines, they actually work together in harmony to advance your fitness goals. Cardiovascular exercises prepare the body to burn calories, elevate mood, and improve cardiovascular health. Strength exercise, meanwhile, tones your muscles, strengthens your bones, and speeds up your metabolism.

These two types of exercise combine into one seamless workout regimen when it is well-balanced. Include aerobic exercises three to five times a week, switching between steady-state cardio and high-intensity interval training (HIIT) workouts. Add two to three days of strength training to this, being sure to work different muscle groups throughout each session. The end result is a thorough regimen that not only supports your goals for weight loss but also improves your general fitness.

Daily Movement: The Quiet Catalyst

It's simple to miss ordinary movement, the unsung hero of fitness, among planned workouts. This includes all of the seemingly unimportant things you do during the day, such taking the stairs, strolling, gardening, and playing with your kids or pets. These activities help you burn calories each day and promote an active lifestyle that will assist your fitness objectives.

Make it a habit to move throughout the day by setting goals like completing a certain number of steps or allotting a certain amount of time to standing. Take quick breaks to stretch or go for a quick stroll, especially if you find yourself spending a lot of time sitting down. Accepting regular movement is a technique to improve your weight loss efforts as well as your joint mobility, blood flow, and general vigor.

Building a Positive Exercise Relationship: Mindset Matters

Exercise has advantages for mental and emotional development in addition to its physical advantages. Exercise is a chance for self-discovery, empowerment, and development rather than a punishment. Change your mindset so that you embrace exercise as an investment in your wellbeing rather than seeing it as a chore. Exercise becomes less of a chore and more of a celebration of your body's potential thanks to this mentality change.

Develop a mindset that values consistency above perfection. Recognise that every workout, no matter its duration or difficulty, helps you advance. Set attainable objectives and acknowledge each success, whether it's logging an additional mile or mastering a challenging yoga position. By incorporating optimism and self-compassion into your fitness routine, you're not only building a stronger body but also cultivating a better relationship with yourself.

The Transforming Empowerment

You are going on a transformative journey as you navigate the worlds of fitness and exercise that goes beyond weight reduction. Your exercise routine is a dynamic journey that reshapes your body, mind, and soul, not just a series of exercises. self can sculpt a stronger, more vibrant self by creating a thorough workout plan that incorporates both cardiovascular and strength training, embracing everyday movement, and cultivating a good exercise mindset.

Exercise is your constant companion as you journey through the next chapters, learning about attitude, healthy behaviors, and methods for long-term maintenance. It is more than just a weight-loss tool; it opens the door to empowerment and a life full of vigor. By embracing exercise, you're embracing the very essence of change—a change that goes far beyond your outward appearance and envelops your entire being in a tapestry of strength, resilience, and wellbeing.

Chapter 4

MINDSET MATTERS

The topography of your mind has incredible influence in the vast panorama of your weight reduction quest. In addition to supporting your physical efforts, having a resilient and upbeat mindset serves as the foundation for your development. This chapter explores the complex world of mindset and how it affects your path within. You'll find the tools that enable you to navigate the inner landscape and harness its potential for long-lasting development, from creating intentional intents to accepting challenges, cultivating self-compassion, and framing setbacks as stepping stones.

Setting Intentions with Purpose: The Leading Light

Your route to a healthier weight starts with a clear intention—a lighthouse that paves the way and strengthens your resolve. Beyond only losing weight, purposeful aspirations also include holistic wellbeing, better energy, improved confidence, and general vigor. Even in the face of difficulties, your actions and decisions are guided by these intentions.

Create your intentions with accuracy and sincerity. Consider more expansive goals like feeling more energized, fitting into a favorite clothing, or accomplishing a physical achievement you've always wanted to do rather than focusing simply on losing weight. Your journey will be fueled by your intentions, which will also serve as a reminder of the significant change you want to experience.

Taking on Challenges: Engines for Growth

Challenges are stepping stones for your growth, not obstacles. Consider challenges as chances to increase your ability for resilience and adaptation rather than as something to be feared. The lessons you learn through challenges help to mold your character and teach you how to negotiate the complex terrain of your path.

Adopt a growth mindset when confronted with a setback or an obstacle that seems insurmountable. Accept the idea that obstacles are not failures, but rather a path to success. Utilize setbacks as opportunities for introspection, education, and recalibrating. You'll find that obstacles hold the secret to your personal development if you approach them with a sense of inquiry and tenacity.

Developing Self-Compassion: Your Inner Haven

Remember to be kind to yourself while you're on your path. The soft response to self-criticism is self-compassion. It entails accepting your flaws and challenges without passing judgment and treating yourself with the same empathy you would a friend.

Use self-compassion when you experience setbacks or times of self-doubt. Offer yourself tolerance and empathy rather than criticizing yourself. Remind yourself that setbacks are a necessary part of the trip and that you are doing the best you can with the tools at your disposal. You can increase emotional resilience and a strong sense of wellbeing by practicing self-compassion.

Setting Backs in the Right Perspective

Reversals do not indicate failure; rather, they present chances for improvement. View losses as brief difficulties that present priceless lessons rather than internalizing them as irreversible defeats. Consider the lessons you've gained from each failure and utilize them to improve your tactics.

Be sure to see setbacks from a growth perspective. Accept them as essential components of your path rather than allowing them to weaken your confidence. By viewing setbacks as stepping stones, you can turn difficult times into sources of resiliency and achievement. Your journey turns into a constant learning and improvement process.

The Influence of Confident Statements

Your thoughts affect your emotions and behavior because they shape your world. Utilizing the strength of affirmations—good phrases that support your ideas and aspirations—can help you develop a positive mindset. Your motivation and self-efficacy will rise as a result of affirmations, which change your ideas to be more positive.

Create affirmations that speak to your desires and goals. Instead of thinking, "I can't resist unhealthy foods," change your thinking to, "I choose to nourish my body with foods that support my well-being." Make a habit of daily repetition of these affirmations. As a result, you develop a positive mindset that helps you move closer to your objectives.

Celebrating achievements and progress

Despite the difficulties, successes frequently go unrecognized. Celebrating your victories and achievements is essential to staying motivated and being recognised for your work. Recognise your accomplishments big and small because they all contribute to the overall picture of your path.

Establish a reward system that supports your goals. Choose experiences or things that improve your well-being instead of food for these rewards. These occasions serve as a reminder of your tenacity and dedication. You may maintain the sensation of accomplishment that drives your momentum by acknowledging your victories.

How to Develop a Transformational Mindset

Recognise that your mindset is the cornerstone of transformation as you navigate the landscape of your weight reduction journey. You may intentionally and purposefully direct the direction of your path by cultivating a resilient and optimistic mindset. Your attitude is the internal compass that directs your path, from setting empowering aspirations and accepting obstacles to cultivating self-compassion and viewing setbacks as stepping stones.

Remember that your mentality continues to be your most effective tool as you explore healthy behaviors, techniques for maintenance, and the conclusion of your transformation as you progress through the next chapters. You may give yourself the tools you need for long-lasting change—change that permeates every aspect of your life and extends beyond your outward appearance—by creating a mentality of growth, positivity, and self-compassion. Take advantage of the influence of your mentality and let it lead you to a future filled with vitality, resiliency, and self-empowerment.

Chapter 5

HEALTHY HABITS FOR LIFE

Long-lasting habits are more important as your weight loss journey advances than quick fixes. Sustainable transformation is cultivating a lifestyle that nurtures your body, mind, and spirit, not fast cures. In this chapter, we explore the topic of healthy habits and how to develop routines that will help your long-term wellbeing. You'll learn the secrets to creating a life bursting with vitality and continuous transformation, from mindful eating to prioritizing sleep, handling stress, staying hydrated, and fostering social connections.

Savoring each bite while eating mindfully

A transforming practice, mindful eating teaches you to appreciate each bite and re-establish a connection with the act of feeding your body. It involves being aware of your hunger signals, eating mindfully, and savouring the flavours and textures of your meal. You're more likely to enjoy your meals, know when you're full, and make deliberate decisions that support your goals if you practice mindful eating.

Remove any distractions from the dining experience to practise mindful eating. Enjoy every bite, paying attention to the flavor, aroma, and texture. Pay attention to your body's cues for hunger and satisfaction, and eat only until you feel completely satisfied. This routine develops a stronger understanding of your body's requirements over time and aids in controlling your appetite.

Sleeping First: The Foundation of Wellness

Sleep is an essential component of good health, not merely a luxury. By controlling hunger hormones, encouraging muscle regeneration, and improving cognitive function, quality sleep helps people lose weight. To maximise your body's restorative functions, aim for 7-9 hours of unbroken sleep each night.

Establish a regular sleep schedule by going to bed and waking up at the same times every day to enhance the quality of your sleep. Establish a relaxing night routine that incorporates pastimes like reading, light stretching, or meditation. To encourage restful sleep, keep your bedroom cold, dark, and comfy. Making sleep a priority is an investment in your health that will pay off in many areas of your life.

Stress management: fostering inner tranquilly

Stress can thwart your attempts to lose weight by inducing emotional eating and messing with your hormonal balance.

Learning stress-reduction strategies equips you with the strength and composure needed to face obstacles in life. Take part in enjoyable pursuits, such as yoga, meditation, journaling, or time spent outdoors.

To center oneself in the now when under stress, try deep breathing or mindfulness techniques. Develop techniques to manage or reduce stressors that you have control over. Keep in mind that stress management is a lifelong skill that benefits both your weight reduction efforts and general wellbeing.

Keep Hydrated by Meeting Your Body's Needs

The foundation of health and vigor is hydration. Digestion, metabolism, and cellular function all depend on water. It is simpler to manage your caloric intake when you drink enough water to keep your appetite under control.

Aim to consume 8 glasses (or about 2 liters) of water each day. Bring a reusable water bottle with you so that you can stay hydrated. For more flavor, add fresh fruits, herbs, or a squeeze of citrus to your water. Develop the habit of drinking water frequently throughout the day and pay attention to your body's thirst signals.

Building Social Bonds: The Influence of Community

The people we hang out with can frequently support healthy behaviours. Maintaining social relationships not only improves your emotional health but also has a favourable impact on your lifestyle decisions. Spend time with people who support your goals and promote healthy habits, such as your friends and family.

Participate in activities that promote social relationships, whether they be cooking classes, group exercise sessions, or just spending time with loved ones. Sharing your experience with others fosters accountability and a sense of community that makes healthy living more fun and long-lasting.

Gratitude Practise: Promoting Positivity

A transforming practice is practicing gratitude, which helps you turn your attention from what you lack to what you do have. Gratitude increases your general wellbeing and encourages a positive outlook. Reflecting on your blessings on a regular basis might make you feel more pleased and less stressed.

Include acts of thankfulness in your regular routine. Keep a thankfulness diary in which you list three things every day for which you are thankful. Show others your appreciation through pleasant words and deeds. This routine alters your perspective over time, encouraging positivity and an attitude of abundance.

Creating Lifelong Healthy Habits

Recognise that developing healthy habits is the foundation of long-lasting change as you walk the path to transformation. The foundations of a robust and satisfying life are mindful nutrition, making sleep a priority, controlling stress, drinking plenty of water, fostering social relationships, and engaging in acts of appreciation.

Remember that your habits are the threads that weave your daily existence as you proceed through the remaining chapters, learning tactics for upkeep and the completion of your transformation. You may create a life that is full of vitality, resiliency, and long-lasting wellbeing by cultivating these practises. Accept these habits as lifelong practices that will help you on your path to lasting transformation rather than as temporary goals.

Chapter 6

NAVIGATING CHALLENGES

As your journey to lose weight comes to an end, a new chapter—one characterized by maintenance and a commitment to the long-term goal you've created—begins. Maintaining your success is more than just holding on to what you've already accomplished; it's a dynamic process that calls for ongoing commitment, thoughtful decisions, and a persistent mentality. We examine the nuances of maintenance, the skill of overcoming plateaus, setting new objectives, and embracing a lifetime of vibrant well-being in this chapter. In this chapter, your transformation transforms into a way of life and your journey turns into a tapestry woven with tenacity, development, and long-term success.

Honoring Your Progress: The Art of Maintenance

A balanced strategy that maintains your success replaces the intensive focus on weight loss during maintenance. It's evidence of your commitment and support for the new way of life you've developed. While the early phase of weight loss may be characterised by abrupt fluctuations, maintenance places an emphasis on steadiness and homeostasis.

Continue engaging in the healthy routines you've developed—mindful eating, consistent exercise, and self-care—to get through the maintenance phase. Regularly check your weight and measurements to track your progress, and make any necessary dietary or behavioral changes. Accept that variations are normal and a necessary part of the process. Keep in mind that maintenance is a sustained commitment to your wellbeing.

Getting Past Stoppages: The Way to Advancement

Any transformational journey will inevitably experience challenges. Although they could be annoying, they also present chances for improvement. As your body adjusts to changes and seeks homeostasis, plateaus frequently happen. Adopting tactics that revitalize your progress is the key.

Consider changing your training programme or adding new workouts to challenge your body to get through plateaus. Consider your food choices, and see if you need to make any changes. Keep a record of your eating habits and workout routines to spot any trends or areas that require adjustment. Be patient and persistent; plateaus are only temporary, and your commitment will help you go past them.

Setting New Objectives: Continuing the Progress

Setting new goals becomes crucial when you move from weight reduction to maintenance. Whether your goals are focused on personal development, culinary adventures, or physical health, they offer your trip direction and help you go forward. These objectives encourage constant inspiration and enthusiasm.

Create fresh objectives that fit your current stage of the trip. Think about setting goals like running a half-marathon, learning a new nutritious meal every week, or starting daily meditation. These objectives direct your ongoing development and extension and serve as a constant reminder of the lifelong nature of your path.

Choosing to Live Well for a Lifetime

Your journey to losing weight is a first step towards a lifetime of wellbeing. Accept the fact that your transformation is a continuous process that goes beyond simple physical improvements to encompass holistic vitality. Your journey is a tapestry made of tenacity, development, and long-lasting success.

Develop a mindset that sees dedication to wellbeing as a lifetime endeavor. Maintain your good habits, make thoughtful decisions, and look for new growth opportunities. Accept the virtue of adaptability and modify your routines to suit the various stages of life. Stay tuned into your body's signals, congratulate it on its accomplishments, and give it the rest and nutrition it needs.

Your legacy, your journey

Recognise that you've started a transformation that goes beyond weight reduction as you approach maintenance and the next stage of your journey. Your path is proof of your fortitude, perseverance, and unshakable dedication to wellbeing. You're creating a legacy of resiliency and vigorous living by navigating the maintenance phase, getting over plateaus, setting new goals, and embracing lifetime well-being.

Keep in mind that when you progress through the remaining chapters and begin the lifelong adventure of preserving your change, your journey will be a reflection of your inner fortitude and the strength of your decisions. Accept your metamorphosis as it progresses, celebrating each victory and failure. Your journey is more than just a quest for physical improvement; it's a symbol of the resilient spirit you carry, a spirit that overcomes obstacles, welcomes change, and radiates health and vigor for years to come.

Chapter 7

MAINTENANCE AND BEYOND

A new phase of your weight loss journey emerges as you progress, one that goes beyond simple maintenance and into the area of total wellbeing. Beyond the first successes and unwavering dedication, there is a landscape full of opportunity for development, self-discovery, and the nurturing of a fulfilling existence. We explore the harmony of physical, mental, and emotional health, the significance of continual self-care, and the legacy of your transformation as we delve into the complexities of living a life immersed in wellness in this chapter. This is the point at which your transformational experience turns into a legacy of enduring vitality and empowerment.

Health in Balance: Mental, Emotional, and Physical

The goal of your trip isn't only to reach a certain weight; it's to balance all of the aspects of your wellbeing. Your body, mind, and emotions are all intertwined, so it's important to take care of each one if you want to keep making progress.

Take part in regular exercise not just for the physical advantages but also for the positive effects it has on your mood. Take part in enjoyable activities that increase your heart rate and challenge your body. Nurture your mental health by practicing mindfulness through exercises like yoga and meditation. Recognise your feelings and work through them, seeking help if necessary. A tapestry of well-being is woven by the harmony of your physical, mental, and emotional health and supports your change.

Continued Self-Care: Feeding Your Soul

An ongoing commitment to put your health first is self-care. It's not a luxury; it's a must that fosters your development and resiliency. Self-care rituals help you maintain equilibrium, tranquility, and vigor in your life.

Develop a collection of self-care techniques that speak to you. Reading, being outside, taking relaxing baths, or engaging in creative activities are some examples of this. Put sleep and relaxation first to restore your vitality. Regularly evaluate your self-care practice and make any adjustments to meet your changing needs. Keep in mind that taking care of yourself shows that you are deserving of love and affection.

Building Supportive Networks and Positive Relationships

Your wellbeing is significantly impacted by the relationships you cultivate. Spend time with people who inspire and raise you up. Develop relationships based on mutual respect, comprehension, and shared principles.

Take part in social gatherings, family outings, or neighborhood events that promote meaningful connections. Seek out those who have similar goals or journeys. Your motivation and dedication to well-being are strengthened by the uplifting energy of helpful relationships.

Taking up New Challenges Is A Lifelong Journey

Your transition has come to a close, yet this is just the beginning of another story. Accept new challenges that fit your changing objectives. These difficulties support your development, vigor, and feeling of direction.

Set goals that are in line with your path, such as a new fitness objective, a charitable undertaking, or the acquisition of a new talent. Every difficulty is a chance to push your boundaries, find untapped strengths, and keep growing. As long as you're willing to learn and explore new things, your path will remain active.

Making a Transformational Legacy

Your transformational journey is more than a purely individual endeavor; it leaves a lasting impact on both your life and the lives of people around you. Your personal transformation serves as motivation for others to accept change and put their health first.

Honesty and openness are key when sharing your experiences. Talk about the difficulties you overcame, your personal development, and the enduring effects on your life. Your experience inspires others to set out on their own transformative journeys by acting as a beacon of hope and resiliency. Your beneficial impact on others will serve as your legacy in addition to your own personal growth.

A Life Unveiled

You should be aware that your trip is a complex voyage into vigorous living as you stand on the edge of well-being that goes beyond upkeep. You may create a life of deep meaning and enduring wellness by balancing your physical, mental, and emotional well-being, prioritizing self-care, cultivating strong connections, accepting new challenges, and leaving a legacy of transformation.

Remember that your transformation is a symphony of resilience, strength, and authenticity as you move forward, exploring the road of continued well-being and the lasting legacy you're creating. Accept the limitless potential of your life as it has been revealed—a life bursting with vitality, empowerment, and the significant contribution you were meant to make to the world.

Chapter 8

RECIPES AND MEAL PLANS

The notes of nutrition are an essential part of the big symphony that is your weight loss journey. This chapter digs into the world of wholesome dishes and meal planning, revealing a flavor palette that supports your objectives. We study the art of preparing meals that fuel your transformation, from wholesome breakfasts to filling lunches and delectable feasts. These dishes are a celebration of flavor, energy, and the adventure you've traveled; they go beyond providing food for survival.

Putting Together a Balanced Plate: The Basis of Nutrition

The evidence of mindful eating and providing your body with a range of nutrients is a balanced plate. A typical meal should include a well-balanced mix of proteins, carbs, good fats, and a wide variety of veggies.

Create your plate with purpose: split it in half between colorful veggies, lean proteins, and entire grains, along with some healthy fats. This harmony promotes steady energy levels, satiety, and general health.

The Morning Boost breakfast

Breakfast is a chance to start the day on a positive note and with vigor. To stay full and focused, choose foods high in protein and fiber.

Consider a filling bowl of muesli with nuts, seeds and berries on top. Eat some eggs scrambled with spinach and some whole-grain bread. These breakfast options create a good mood for the day.

Wholesome Lunch and Dinner Recipes

Lunch: An Indulgent Midday Break

Your lunchtime fuel, lunch will keep you going through the afternoon. Select dishes that feature a variety of veggies, lean proteins, and complex carbohydrates.

Take pleasure in a salad that includes grilled chicken, chickpeas, mixed greens, and a rainbow of colorful vegetables. For a delicious portable treat, wrap turkey and avocado in a whole-grain tortilla. These lunch options meet your nutritional demands while also pleasing to the palate.

Culinary Delights for dinner

The chance to unwind and enjoy the flavors of the day is at dinner. Accept meals that are a feast for the senses in addition to being nourishing.

Prepare quinoa and simmer asparagus to go with a baked salmon filet. Enjoy a brown rice and tofu stir-fry with vegetables. These meal selections are the perfect example of how taste and health can coexist.

Smart Snacking Options

In-between-meal sustenance is provided by snacks. Select foods that are filling and high in nutrients.

Grab a handful of mixed nuts and dried fruit to munch on. Grass-topped Greek yogurt is delicious with honey drizzled over it. These snacks help you stay energized and satisfy cravings.

Hydration: A Crucial Ingredient

Vitality is built on hydration. Water, herbal teas, and naturally flavored drinks should be consumed throughout the day.

Carry a reusable water bottle, and make it a point to stay hydrated all day. Drink herbal teas to relax and refresh. The simplest method to boost your general wellbeing is to stay hydrated.

Meal Preparation: A Guide to Success

Your transformation journey's hidden weapon is meal planning. It provides order, practicality, and a safeguard against rash decisions.

Every week, set some time to plan your meals and make a shopping list. Prepare recipes that can be portioned and kept for later use in large batches. Making nourishing decisions even on hectic days is ensured by having meals on hand.

The Art of Nourishment

A celebration of your journey and an act of self-care, nourishing your body. Always keep in mind that each bite is a stroke on the canvas of your transformation as you go through the recipes and meal plans in this chapter. Your symphony of vigor and wellbeing is a result of the flavors and nutrients you enjoy.

Recognise that you are nourishing not just your body but also your spirit as you travel forward, experimenting with these dishes and adding them into your meal planning. Accept the art of food as a crucial component of your transformational path—a journey that takes into account both your bodily and spiritual well-being.

Chapter 9

SUCCESS STORIES

Although every path is distinct, transformation runs through them all. This chapter is a tapestry made of motivating triumph stories, a celebration of people who have accepted change, persisted through difficulties, and come out on top. These tales serve as an example of the strength of tenacity, grit, and the unyielding human spirit. May these stories encourage you, reaffirm your own journey, and serve as a helpful reminder that you have the power to transform.

Real-Life Transformations

Richard Transformation: From Struggle to Victory

Richard's journey started with the realization that, due to the demands of his busy life, his health had suffered. He decided to take control of his well being once more and started down a transformative road. He developed healthy behaviors that progressively brought about deep change with perseverance and the assistance of a caring community.

Richard lost weight and increased vitality via regular exercise, thoughtful eating, and unshakable devotion. His narrative serves as a monument to both the amazing power of simple, regular actions and the resiliency of the human spirit. The trip itself—the growth, the setbacks, and the victories—is what transforms us, not simply the final goal, as Richard's story reminds us.

A Breakthrough: Jane's Empowerment

The narrative of Jane is one of overcoming obstacles and discovering inner strength. She struggled with body image issues and self-doubt, which prevented her from pursuing her aspirations. But Jane made the decision that she wouldn't let her fear keep her from doing things.

Jane changed her perspective by using courage as her compass. She fed her body with healthy meals, engaged in empowering activities, and surrounded herself with inspiring people. The transformational potential of self-love and the reverberating effects it may have on all facets of life are best demonstrated by Jane's path. Her experience shows us that the path to empowerment and self-discovery is a strong force that can tear down the barriers to self-limitation.

Maria's Renewal: A Healing Journey

Maria's path to change was one of recovery and regeneration. She struggled with health concerns and realized she needed nurturing and care for her wellbeing. Maria started a comprehensive healing journey that included mental, emotional, and physical recovery.

Maria's body started to heal and her spirit was revived via yoga, meditation, and healthy foods. Her experience serves as a reminder that transformation involves more than just physical changes; it also entails embracing self-compassion and placing a high priority on self-care. Because it supports the body, mind, and spirit, seeking wellness is a profound act of love, as Maria's journey shows us.

The Resilient Spirit: Mark's Victory Over Difficulties

In spite of difficulties, Mark's transformational journey was characterized by resilience. He struggled with disappointments, wounds, and self-doubt. But Mark refused to let his struggles define him; instead, he saw them as opportunities for personal development.

Mark conquered challenges that looked impossible with the help of his loved ones and his everlasting commitment. His experience serves as a monument to the strength of tenacity and the unwavering human spirit. Mark's experience serves as a reminder that while the path to transformation may be difficult, our success is determined by the strength we muster.

Lessons Learned from Others' Journeys

Each success story is a thread in the overall transformational tapestry. Remember that your journey is woven into this tapestry, an evolving tale of empowerment, progress, and resiliency, as you read these stories. Accept the lessons these tales have to teach you about the value of self-love, the strength of will, and the grace of accepting change.

Your path has been singular, and your tale is just waiting to be told. Make use of these triumphant stories as motivation as you continue on your road. Let them serve as a reminder to you that transformation is an ongoing process that affects both your physical and spiritual well-being and leads to a life of vibrant wellbeing.

CONCLUSION

Consider the symphony of change that has developed within you as you approach the last chapter of this transforming journey. You've set out on a significant journey, one that is characterized by growth, resilience, and the unwavering pursuit of a fulfilling life, starting from the initial spark of motivation and ending with the unflinching commitment to well-being. The strands of your trip are brought together in this finale, which also offers insights on the path you've taken and the opportunities that lay ahead.

A Self-Discovery Journey

Your transformation path involves much more than just bodily changes. It's been a journey of self-discovery—an investigation of your innate talents, interests, and resiliency. You've discovered reserves of tenacity with each difficulty you've encountered that you might not have realised existed. Accept these discoveries with open arms because they represent the real rewards of your trip.

The Power of Repetition

Your compass has been consistency throughout this voyage. It involves making a daily commitment to eating good foods, exercising, and taking care of your overall well being. Your unwavering commitment has demonstrated that change is not brought about by a few large gestures but rather by a series of modest yet persistent activities. Keep in mind that every action you've performed has helped you succeed.

Being Resilient in the Face of Difficulties

Your challenges have been your teachers, helping you to develop and become more independent. You have shown great resilience, whether it was in navigating plateaus, overcoming setbacks, or dealing with self-doubt. These difficulties weren't obstacles; they were chances to expand your horizons, change your perspective, and become more resilient than before.

The Magnificence of Self-Care

Your journey has been built on self-care, which is evidence of your deservingness of love and nurture. Your body and soul have both benefited from the practices you've adopted. You've drawn a picture of a life bursting with vitality and well-being through mindfulness, gratitude, and the development of meaningful relationships.

A Tradition of Empowerment

Your journey is a lasting legacy that inspires and empowers others. Remember that you are impacting individuals in your immediate vicinity as you continue to cultivate your development. Your commitment, tenacity, and love of yourself serve as lights that direct others towards their own transforming journeys. Since your experience has the potential to inspire change in others, be honest when sharing your path.

Celebrating Your Achievements

As you finish this chapter, keep in mind that your journey is a lifelong adventure that extends beyond these pages. With an open mind and a sense of wonder, embrace the opportunities that lie ahead. The road may keep changing, but your dedication to your wellbeing never wavers.

Celebrate each accomplishment and understand that your transformation is a continual symphony that balances your physical, mental, and spiritual well-being. Embrace each step of your path because it adds to the fabric of your life, which displays your bravery, tenacity, and extraordinary potential.

Looking Ahead: A Healthier Future

Keep in mind that your transformation is a living artwork as you conclude this chapter and move into the world beyond these words. It is a physical representation of your dedication to self-improvement, resiliency in the face of difficulties, and acceptance of change. Your path is a tribute to your fortitude, spirit, and unrelenting pursuit of a life rich in vitality, happiness, and the delight of change. Your journey is evidence of the extraordinary person you are—someone who has spun a tapestry of change that will continue to motivate and inspire people for years to come.